THE UNTOLD BATTLE AGAINST BREAST CANCER

Discover the Courage, Decisions, and Triumphs Behind Olivia Munn's Inspiring Journey Through Diagnosis, Treatment, and Advocacy.

David L. Ellington

Copyright © , 2024

All rights reserved. No part of this publication may be reproduced, distributed, or transmitted in any form or by any means, including photocopying, recording, or other electronic or mechanical methods, without the prior written permission of the publisher, except in the case of brief quotations embodied in critical reviews and certain other non-commercial uses permitted by copyright law.

Table of Content

Introduction

Chapter 1: A Surprise Diagnosis

Chapter 2: Understanding the Risk Factors

Chapter 3: Facing the Reality

Chapter 4: Making Informed Decisions

Chapter 5: Finding Strength in Vulnerability

Chapter 6: Advocating for Awareness

Chapter 7: Navigating Life After Cancer

Chapter 8: Empowering Others

Chapter 9: Messages of Hope and Gratitude

Conclusion: A Call to Action

Introduction

Olivia Munn, celebrated for her roles in "The Newsroom" and "X-Men: Apocalypse," has long been a beacon of strength and resilience in the entertainment industry. Her infectious smile and magnetic charisma have endeared her to millions around the world. Yet, behind the glamour of Hollywood lies a deeply personal journey—one marked by unexpected twists and profound challenges.

In March 2024, Olivia Munn made headlines not for her latest film or television project, but for a revelation that would send shockwaves through her fanbase and beyond. With unwavering courage and transparency, Munn took to social media to share a deeply personal chapter of her life—a journey marked by resilience, vulnerability, and unwavering determination.

The revelation began with a simple yet life-altering event—a routine mammogram. Like many women, Munn approached the appointment with a sense of duty and responsibility to her health. Little did she know that this seemingly ordinary check-up would set off a chain of events that would redefine her life in ways she never imagined.

Following the mammogram, Munn's journey took an unexpected turn when her OB-GYN made a crucial decision—to calculate her breast cancer risk assessment score. It was a decision that would ultimately prove to be life-saving. Despite Munn's initial reservations, this proactive approach to healthcare would soon reveal a startling truth—she was facing a formidable opponent in the form of breast cancer.

For Munn, the diagnosis came as a thunderbolt from the clear blue sky—a stark reminder of life's unpredictability and the fragility of human existence. In the blink of an eye, the world as she knew it was turned upside down, and she found herself grappling with emotions ranging from shock and disbelief to fear and uncertainty.

Yet, amidst the whirlwind of emotions, Munn's unwavering spirit shone through. Rather than succumbing to despair, she made a conscious choice—a choice to confront her diagnosis head-on and to navigate the turbulent waters of cancer with courage and grace.

As Munn candidly shared in her Instagram post, her journey over the past ten months has been marked by countless surgeries, days spent in bed, and a relentless pursuit of knowledge about cancer and its treatment. It has been a journey filled with highs and lows, triumphs and setbacks, but through it all, Munn has remained steadfast in her resolve to emerge stronger and more resilient than ever before.

What makes Munn's journey all the more remarkable is her unwavering determination to turn adversity into an opportunity for growth and empowerment. Rather than retreating into the shadows, she has chosen to shine a spotlight on her experience—not for the sake of fame or attention, but as a beacon of hope and inspiration for others facing similar battles.

Indeed, Munn's decision to share her story publicly was not made lightly. It was a decision borne out of a deep sense of responsibility—to herself, to her loved ones, and to the countless individuals around the world who may find solace and strength in her words.

As she eloquently expressed in her Instagram post, Munn's journey is not just her own—it is a testament to the resilience of the human spirit, the power of community, and the transformative potential of adversity. It is a reminder that even in our darkest moments, we possess within us the strength to rise above our circumstances and emerge victorious.

In the pages that follow, we will delve deeper into Olivia Munn's courageous journey—a journey marked by resilience, vulnerability, and unwavering determination. We will explore the challenges she faced, the lessons she learned, and the profound impact her story has had on countless individuals around the world.

But above all, we will celebrate the indomitable spirit of Olivia Munn—a woman who, in the face of adversity, chose not to be defined by her circumstances, but rather to rise above them with courage, grace, and unyielding hope. Join us as we embark on a journey of inspiration, empowerment, and above all, resilience.

Chapter 1: A Surprise Diagnosis

In the vast tapestry of life, there are moments that stand out, moments that redefine our understanding of ourselves and the world around us. For Olivia Munn, one such moment came unexpectedly, altering the trajectory of her life in ways she could never have imagined. It was a moment that underscored the importance of vigilance, of listening to one's body, and of the critical role that early detection plays in the fight against breast cancer.

In her Instagram post on that fateful Wednesday, Olivia Munn bravely shared her journey with the world. She recounted the shock of receiving a breast cancer diagnosis, a diagnosis that blindsided her despite her outward appearance of health. It was a stark reminder that cancer does not discriminate, that it can strike anyone, regardless of age, fame, or fortune.

As Munn reflected on her journey, she emphasized the crucial role that routine screenings play in detecting breast cancer at its earliest stages. She recounted how a simple mammogram, a routine procedure recommended for women over a certain age or with certain risk factors, led to the discovery of her cancer. It was a testament to the power of preventive healthcare, of taking proactive steps to safeguard one's well-being.

Breast cancer screenings, such as mammograms, are essential tools in the arsenal against this insidious disease. They allow healthcare providers to detect abnormalities in breast tissue long before they manifest as symptoms, increasing the likelihood of successful treatment and recovery. Yet, despite their importance, screenings are often overlooked or postponed due to fear, uncertainty, or simply the busyness of life.

Munn's experience serves as a poignant reminder of the significance of early detection. Had she not undergone that routine mammogram, her cancer may have gone undetected until it was too late. It highlights the need for women of all ages to prioritize their breast health, to schedule regular screenings as part of their healthcare regimen.

But routine screenings are only one piece of the puzzle. In Munn's case, it was her breast cancer risk assessment score that ultimately led to her diagnosis. This score, calculated by her OB-GYN based on factors such as age, familial history, and genetic predisposition, identified her as a high-risk individual deserving of further scrutiny. It was a pivotal moment, a turning point in her journey toward diagnosis and treatment.

Breast cancer risk assessment is a valuable tool in identifying individuals who may be at increased risk of developing the disease. By taking into account factors such as family history, genetic mutations, and personal health history, healthcare providers can better tailor screening and prevention strategies to individual patients. It empowers individuals to take control of their health, to make informed decisions about their care, and to advocate for themselves within the healthcare system.

For Munn, her risk assessment score served as a lifeline, a beacon of hope in the midst of uncertainty. It prompted further testing, leading to the early detection of her cancer and ultimately to life-saving treatment. It underscores the importance of personalized medicine, of treating each patient as an individual with unique needs and circumstances.

As we embark on this journey with Olivia Munn, let us heed the lessons of her experience. Let us prioritize our health, our well-being, and the well-being of those we love. Let us not wait for symptoms to manifest or for fear to paralyze us into inaction. Instead, let us embrace the power of early detection, of routine screenings, and of personalized healthcare. For in doing so, we honor not only ourselves but all those who have walked this path before us.

Chapter 2: Understanding the Risk Factors

Breast cancer is a complex disease influenced by a multitude of factors, both genetic and environmental. In this chapter, we will delve into the various risk factors associated with breast cancer, shedding light on the importance of understanding these factors for early detection and prevention. We will also explore Olivia Munn's personal experience with genetic testing and the significance of negative results in her journey.

The Multifaceted Nature of Breast Cancer Risk

Breast cancer risk factors can be broadly categorized into two main types: non-modifiable and modifiable. Non-modifiable risk factors are those that cannot be changed, such as age, gender, and family history. Modifiable risk factors, on the other hand, are those that can be influenced by lifestyle choices and environmental factors, such as diet, physical activity, and alcohol consumption.

Age

Age is one of the most significant risk factors for breast cancer. The risk of developing breast cancer increases with age, with the majority of cases diagnosed in women over the age of 50. However, it's important to note that breast cancer can occur at any age, and younger women are not immune to the disease.

Familial History

A family history of breast cancer can significantly increase an individual's risk of developing the disease. Women with a first-degree relative (such as a mother, sister, or daughter) who has been diagnosed with breast cancer have a higher risk than those with no family history. Additionally, having multiple relatives affected by breast cancer or a history of breast cancer in male relatives can further elevate the risk.

Genetic Predisposition

Certain genetic mutations can predispose individuals to breast cancer. The most well-known of these mutations is the BRCA gene mutation, which significantly increases the risk of both breast and ovarian cancer. Other genetic mutations, such as those associated with Lynch syndrome and Li-Fraumeni syndrome, can also increase breast cancer risk. However, it's important to recognize that the majority of breast cancer cases are not due to inherited genetic mutations but rather occur sporadically.

Olivia Munn's Journey with Genetic Testing

In her journey with breast cancer, Olivia Munn underwent genetic testing to assess her risk of carrying genetic mutations associated with the disease. Genetic testing involves analyzing a sample of blood or saliva to identify specific mutations in genes known to be associated with cancer.

Munn's decision to undergo genetic testing was influenced by her family history and her desire to gain a better understanding of her personal risk profile. Despite testing negative for mutations in genes associated with breast cancer, including the BRCA gene, Munn's journey underscores the importance of comprehensive risk assessment beyond genetic testing alone.

The Significance of Negative Results

For individuals like Olivia Munn who test negative for known genetic mutations, the absence of a positive result may provide a sense of relief. However, it's essential to recognize that genetic testing only captures a portion of the overall risk profile for breast cancer.

Negative results do not guarantee immunity from the disease, as the majority of breast cancer cases are not attributed to inherited genetic mutations. Other risk factors, such as age, lifestyle choices, and environmental exposures, also play a significant role in breast cancer development.

Empowering Knowledge for Prevention

Understanding the various risk factors associated with breast cancer empowers individuals to take proactive steps towards prevention and early detection. While certain risk factors, such as age and family history, cannot be changed, lifestyle modifications, such as maintaining a healthy weight, engaging in regular physical activity, and limiting alcohol consumption, can help reduce the risk of developing breast cancer.

Chapter 3: Facing the Reality

Facing the reality of a breast cancer diagnosis is an emotional journey filled with uncertainty, fear, and a myriad of conflicting emotions. For Olivia Munn, learning about her diagnosis was a seismic event that upended her life and forced her to confront the harsh reality of her situation. In this chapter, we delve into Munn's emotional rollercoaster upon receiving the life-altering news, her initial reactions, and the profound process of coming to terms with her diagnosis. Moreover, we shine a light on the invaluable role played by her loved ones in providing unwavering support during her darkest moments.

The moment Munn received the diagnosis, it felt as if the ground beneath her feet had crumbled away, leaving her suspended in a whirlwind of disbelief and shock. Like many who face such devastating news, her mind raced with questions and uncertainties, grappling with the overwhelming weight of what lay ahead. The fear of the unknown loomed large, casting a shadow over her thoughts and emotions. How would she navigate the complexities of treatment? What would the future hold for her and her loved ones? These questions swirled relentlessly in her mind, threatening to consume her with anxiety and despair.

Initially, Munn's reactions were a tumultuous mix of disbelief, anger, and profound sadness. The news felt surreal, as if she were living in a nightmare from which she couldn't wake up. She struggled to comprehend the gravity of her diagnosis, wrestling with feelings of denial and disbelief. As the reality of her situation began to sink in, waves of fear and anxiety washed over her, threatening to drown her in a sea of despair. The future she had envisioned suddenly felt uncertain and precarious, shattering her sense of security and stability.

Coming to terms with her diagnosis was a gradual and arduous process for Munn, marked by moments of profound introspection and soul-searching. She had to confront her deepest fears and insecurities, summoning the courage to confront the harsh realities of her situation head-on. It was a journey fraught with pain and uncertainty, yet it was also a journey of profound self-discovery and resilience.

With the unwavering support of her loved ones, Munn found the strength to face her diagnosis with courage and grace. Her family, friends, and partner rallied around her, offering a steady anchor amidst the storm of emotions. Their presence was a source of comfort and solace, providing a glimmer of hope in her darkest moments. Their unwavering love and support served as a lifeline, helping her navigate the turbulent waters of her diagnosis with courage and resilience.

The importance of support from loved ones during difficult times cannot be overstated. For Munn, the outpouring of love and support from her family and friends was a source of strength and inspiration, helping her find the courage to confront her diagnosis with resilience and determination. Their unwavering presence served as a reminder that she was not alone in her journey, that there were people who loved her and stood by her side no matter what.

In the crucible of adversity, Munn discovered the true power of love and solidarity, finding solace in the embrace of her loved ones. Their unwavering support helped her navigate the darkest moments of her journey, offering a beacon of hope amidst the storm. In their love and presence, she found the courage to face her diagnosis with grace and resilience, emerging stronger and more resilient than ever before.

Chapter 4: Making Informed Decisions

Olivia Munn's journey through breast cancer was marked by a proactive approach to treatment, driven by a desire to confront the disease head-on and regain control over her health. In this chapter, we delve into Munn's decision-making process regarding treatment options, particularly focusing on her choice to undergo surgeries and a mastectomy. Additionally, we explore the significance of Luminal B breast cancer, its aggressive nature, and the considerations involved in selecting the most effective treatment plans.

From the moment Munn received her breast cancer diagnosis, she embarked on a mission to gather as much information as possible about her condition and available treatment options. Armed with knowledge and supported by her medical team, Munn navigated the complex landscape of cancer treatment with determination and resilience.

One of the pivotal decisions Munn faced was whether to undergo surgeries, including a mastectomy, as part of her treatment plan. Despite the daunting prospect of surgical intervention, Munn approached this option with a pragmatic mindset, weighing the potential benefits against the associated risks. Ultimately, she recognized that surgery offered the best chance of removing the cancerous tissue and reducing the risk of recurrence. Moreover, opting for a double mastectomy provided Munn with a sense of empowerment, allowing her to take proactive steps to safeguard her health and minimize the likelihood of future complications.

The significance of Luminal B breast cancer cannot be overstated in Munn's treatment journey. Luminal B tumors are characterized by their aggressive nature and rapid growth, posing significant challenges for both patients and healthcare providers. Unlike less aggressive forms of breast cancer, Luminal B tumors require prompt and decisive intervention to prevent the disease from spreading and metastasizing to other parts of the body. Understanding the unique characteristics of her cancer subtype empowered Munn to make informed decisions about her treatment plan, ensuring that she received the most effective care tailored to her specific needs.

In the process of making informed decisions about her treatment, Munn relied on the expertise of her medical team and sought guidance from trusted healthcare professionals. Consulting with oncologists, surgeons, and other specialists enabled Munn to gain valuable insights into the potential benefits and risks of various treatment modalities, allowing her to make choices aligned with her health goals and preferences. Moreover, Munn actively engaged in discussions with her healthcare providers, asking questions, expressing concerns, and advocating for her own well-being throughout the decision-making process.

The decision to undergo surgeries and a mastectomy was not made lightly but was rooted in Munn's unwavering commitment to her health and future well-being. By choosing to confront her cancer with courage and resolve, Munn demonstrated resilience in the face of adversity and served as an inspiration to others navigating similar challenges. Her proactive approach to treatment exemplifies the importance of taking an active role in one's healthcare journey, advocating for personalized care and making decisions based on sound medical advice and individual circumstances.

Chapter 5: Finding Strength in Vulnerability

Olivia Munn's journey through breast cancer was not just about battling physical challenges but also navigating the emotional rollercoaster that comes with such a diagnosis. In this chapter, we delve into Munn's reflections on vulnerability and resilience, her coping mechanisms, and the importance of self-care and support from others.

Throughout her journey, Munn found herself confronting vulnerability in ways she never imagined. The initial shock of the diagnosis left her feeling raw and exposed, as if the ground had been pulled from beneath her feet. Yet, in the midst of uncertainty, she discovered a newfound strength in embracing vulnerability. Instead of viewing it as a weakness, she learned to see it as a source of courage and authenticity.

Munn recalls moments when vulnerability became her greatest asset, allowing her to connect with others on a deeper level. Whether it was sharing her fears with loved ones or reaching out for support from fellow survivors, she found solace in the vulnerability of human connection. It was through these moments of openness and honesty that she discovered the true power of resilience.

Coping with the emotional toll of cancer required Munn to develop a toolkit of strategies for maintaining her emotional well-being. One of the most powerful coping mechanisms she found was the practice of mindfulness and meditation. By grounding herself in the present moment, she was able to find moments of peace amidst the chaos of treatment and recovery. Through mindfulness, she learned to cultivate gratitude for the small joys in life, even in the face of adversity.

Another key aspect of Munn's coping strategy was the importance of self-compassion. Instead of berating herself for feeling scared or anxious, she learned to treat herself with kindness and understanding. This meant giving herself permission to rest when she needed it, honoring her emotions without judgment, and practicing self-care in all its forms.

Self-care became an essential part of Munn's healing journey, encompassing everything from physical exercise to creative expression. Whether it was taking long walks in nature, indulging in her favorite hobbies, or simply allowing herself to rest, she made a conscious effort to prioritize her well-being. She discovered the healing power of laughter, surrounding herself with people who lifted her spirits and brought joy into her life.

Yet, perhaps the most transformative aspect of Munn's journey was the support she received from others. From her family and friends to fellow survivors and healthcare professionals, she found strength in the collective embrace of community. Their words of encouragement, acts of kindness, and unwavering presence reminded her that she was never alone in her fight.

Munn emphasizes the importance of reaching out for support when needed, whether it's through therapy, support groups, or simply leaning on loved ones for comfort. She acknowledges that vulnerability can be scary, but it's also where we find our greatest source of strength. By allowing ourselves to be seen and supported, we open ourselves up to a world of healing and possibility.

Chapter 6: Advocating for Awareness

In Chapter 6 of "Navigating Breast Cancer: Olivia Munn's Journey to Resilience," we delve into Olivia Munn's courageous decision to share her personal battle with breast cancer publicly and her efforts to raise awareness about this prevalent disease. Munn's advocacy not only sheds light on the challenges faced by those affected by breast cancer but also highlights the transformative power of celebrity influence in health awareness campaigns.

Olivia Munn's decision to share her breast cancer journey with the world was not made lightly. Like many individuals faced with a life-altering diagnosis, Munn grappled with the initial shock and uncertainty that often accompany such news. However, as she navigated through her treatment and recovery process, Munn recognized the opportunity to use her platform to spark meaningful conversations about breast cancer awareness, early detection, and the importance of proactive healthcare.

For Munn, sharing her story publicly was about more than just personal catharsis; it was a call to action. By opening up about her own experiences, Munn hoped to empower others facing similar challenges, provide support to those in need, and ultimately contribute to the collective effort to combat breast cancer. In doing so, she became a beacon of hope and inspiration for countless individuals around the world.

The impact of celebrity advocacy on health awareness campaigns cannot be overstated. Celebrities like Olivia Munn possess a unique ability to capture public attention and mobilize audiences in ways that traditional awareness campaigns cannot. Their influential status affords them the opportunity to reach millions of people across various platforms, from social media to television interviews and beyond.

When a celebrity like Olivia Munn shares their personal experiences with a health condition like breast cancer, it humanizes the disease and makes it relatable to a wider audience. Suddenly, breast cancer is not just a statistic or a distant concern—it becomes a real and tangible issue that could affect anyone, regardless of fame or fortune. This personal connection fosters empathy and understanding, driving individuals to take action and get involved in the fight against breast cancer.

Moreover, celebrity advocacy helps destigmatize conversations around sensitive topics like cancer and encourages open dialogue within communities. By sharing their stories candidly, celebrities like Olivia Munn help break down barriers and create safe spaces for individuals to discuss their own experiences, seek support, and access resources.

In addition to raising awareness, celebrity advocacy often leads to tangible outcomes in terms of fundraising, research support, and policy changes. Through their influence, celebrities can mobilize their fan bases to donate to charitable organizations, participate in fundraising events, and support initiatives aimed at improving cancer prevention, detection, and treatment.

For readers inspired by Olivia Munn's advocacy efforts, there are numerous ways to get involved in breast cancer awareness initiatives. Local and national organizations dedicated to breast cancer research and support services often welcome volunteers, donors, and advocates. By volunteering your time, participating in fundraising events, or simply spreading awareness within your own community, you can make a meaningful difference in the lives of those affected by breast cancer.

Furthermore, staying informed about breast cancer risk factors, screening guidelines, and available resources is essential for promoting early detection and prevention.

Readers can take proactive steps to prioritize their breast health by scheduling regular screenings, discussing risk factors with their healthcare providers, and advocating for accessible and affordable healthcare options for all.

Chapter 7: Navigating Life After Cancer

Life after cancer treatment marks a new chapter in Olivia Munn's journey, one filled with hope, resilience, and the pursuit of joy. As she emerged from the shadow of cancer, Munn embraced each day with renewed gratitude and a deeper appreciation for life's simple pleasures. In this chapter, we explore Munn's perspective on navigating life after cancer, offering guidance, encouragement, and inspiration for readers facing similar challenges.

Follow-Up Care and Survivorship

Transitioning from active treatment to survivorship can be both exhilarating and daunting. After the intensity of surgeries, chemotherapy, and radiation, survivors often face a new set of challenges, including managing long-term side effects and adjusting to a "new normal." For Olivia Munn, diligent follow-up care became a cornerstone of her post-cancer journey. Regular check-ups with her healthcare team provided reassurance and monitoring of her ongoing health.

Munn emphasizes the importance of staying proactive in one's healthcare journey, advocating for oneself, and seeking support when needed. From scheduling follow-up appointments to monitoring for signs of recurrence, survivors must remain vigilant while also finding balance in their lives.

Embracing Life Post-Treatment

For Munn, embracing life post-treatment meant seizing every opportunity to find joy and meaning in the present moment. Whether it was savoring a quiet morning with her family, immersing herself in creative projects, or simply enjoying the beauty of nature, Munn discovered that happiness could be found in the simplest of experiences.

In the aftermath of cancer, survivors often grapple with a range of emotions, including fear, anxiety, and uncertainty about the future. Munn encourages readers to acknowledge these feelings while also cultivating resilience and optimism. By focusing on the present and cultivating gratitude for each day, survivors can reclaim their lives and find purpose beyond their cancer diagnosis.

Finding Joy in Everyday Moments

Amidst the challenges of survivorship, Munn found solace in the everyday moments that brought her joy. Whether it was sharing laughter with loved ones, pursuing hobbies and interests, or indulging in self-care practices, Munn embraced each day as a gift to be cherished.

For readers navigating life after cancer, Munn offers a message of hope and encouragement. While the road to recovery may be filled with ups and downs, there is beauty to be found in resilience, strength, and the unwavering support of those around us. By focusing on the present moment and finding joy in the journey, survivors can reclaim their lives and move forward with renewed purpose and optimism.

Chapter 8: Empowering Others

Breast cancer is a formidable adversary, but through empowerment and advocacy, individuals can take charge of their health and play an active role in early detection and prevention. In this chapter, we will explore the significance of advocating for one's health, share actionable steps for proactive breast health, and empower readers to become advocates in the fight against breast cancer.

Advocating for One's Health:

Advocating for one's health is a critical component of proactive healthcare. It involves taking ownership of your well-being, seeking out necessary information, and making informed decisions about your health. When it comes to breast cancer, advocacy can mean advocating for regular screenings, understanding risk factors, and advocating for appropriate medical care.

One of the most important aspects of advocacy is communication with healthcare providers. Establishing open and honest communication with your doctor allows you to discuss any concerns or symptoms you may have, as well as to ask questions about recommended screenings and preventative measures. Don't hesitate to advocate for yourself during medical appointments by expressing your preferences, voicing any discomfort or uncertainty, and seeking clarification on medical recommendations.

Additionally, advocating for one's health extends beyond individual actions to broader advocacy efforts within communities and healthcare systems. This can involve supporting policies and initiatives that promote access to affordable healthcare, funding for cancer research, and education on breast health. By advocating for systemic changes, individuals can contribute to improved healthcare outcomes for themselves and others.

Actionable Steps for Proactive Breast Health:

Taking control of your breast health begins with understanding and implementing proactive measures to reduce your risk of breast cancer and detect it early. Here are some actionable steps that readers can take:

> Know Your Risk: Understanding your personal risk factors for breast cancer is essential for making informed decisions about screening and prevention. Factors such as age, family history, genetic mutations, and

lifestyle choices can all influence your risk. Consider discussing your risk factors with a healthcare provider and exploring options for genetic testing if appropriate.

Get Regular Screenings: Routine breast cancer screenings, such as mammograms and clinical breast exams, are crucial for early detection. The American Cancer Society recommends that women aged 40 and older receive annual mammograms, while younger women may benefit from discussing screening options with their doctor based on individual risk factors.

Perform Breast Self-Exams: While not a substitute for mammograms or clinical exams, breast self-exams can help individuals become familiar with their breast tissue and identify any changes or abnormalities. Encourage readers to perform monthly self-exams and to report any concerns to their healthcare provider promptly. Maintain a Healthy Lifestyle: Adopting healthy habits, such as maintaining a balanced diet, engaging in regular exercise, limiting alcohol consumption, and avoiding tobacco products, can help reduce the risk of breast cancer. Encourage readers to prioritize their overall health and well-being through lifestyle choices that support breast health.

Stay Informed: Stay up-to-date on the latest research, guidelines, and recommendations related to breast cancer prevention and screening. Educational resources from reputable organizations like the American Cancer Society, National Cancer Institute, and Susan G. Komen can provide valuable information and support for individuals seeking to proactively manage their breast health.

Empowering Readers as Advocates:

Empowering readers to become advocates for themselves and their loved ones is a powerful tool in the fight against breast cancer. By raising awareness, promoting early detection, and supporting those affected by breast cancer, individuals can make a meaningful impact on their communities and beyond. Here are some ways readers can become advocates:

> Share Your Story: Personal stories have the power to inspire, educate, and raise awareness. Encourage readers to share their experiences with breast cancer, whether as survivors, caregivers, or supporters. By sharing their stories, individuals can break

down stigma, provide encouragement to others, and foster connections within the breast cancer community.

Support Awareness Campaigns: Get involved in breast cancer awareness campaigns and events, such as fundraisers, walks, and community outreach programs. By participating in or volunteering for these initiatives, readers can help raise funds for research, promote early detection, and provide support to those affected by breast cancer.

Advocate for Policy Change: Advocate for policies and legislation that support breast cancer research, access to healthcare, and patient rights. Write to elected officials, join advocacy organizations, and participate in grassroots efforts to influence policy decisions at the local, state, and national levels.

Educate Others: Take on the role of educator by sharing information about breast cancer prevention, screening, and treatment with friends, family members, and community members. Encourage open dialogue about breast health and empower others to take proactive steps towards prevention and early detection.

Support Those in Need: Offer support and encouragement to individuals and families affected by breast cancer. Whether through emotional support, practical assistance, or advocacy efforts, readers can make a difference in the lives of those facing breast cancer by providing a helping hand and a listening ear.

By empowering readers to advocate for their own health and the health of others, we can work together to raise awareness, promote early detection, and ultimately, reduce the impact of breast cancer on individuals and communities worldwide. Through collective action and determination, we can make strides towards a future free from the fear of breast cancer.

Chapter 9: Messages of Hope and Gratitude

In the darkest moments of adversity, messages of hope and gratitude shine like beacons of light, guiding us through the storm. Olivia Munn's journey through breast cancer has been marked not only by her own resilience but also by the unwavering support and love from her cherished friends and family. In this chapter, we delve into the heartfelt messages of hope and gratitude that have illuminated her path, celebrating the collective strength of the breast cancer community and offering words of encouragement to readers embarking on their own journeys of healing and resilience.

Olivia Munn's journey began with a single diagnosis that sent shockwaves through her life. Yet, in the midst of uncertainty and fear, she found herself enveloped in a cocoon of love and support from those closest to her. From her partner, comedian John Mulaney, to her friends and family, the outpouring of messages flooded her with warmth and reassurance.

"I am in awe of your strength and courage," John Mulaney wrote in a heartfelt message to Olivia. "You are a warrior, and I am honored to stand by your side through this journey. Malc and I adore you more than words can express."

These words of love and encouragement echoed throughout Olivia's journey, serving as a constant reminder of the power of human connection in the face of adversity. From handwritten letters to late-night phone calls filled with laughter and tears, each message carried with it a glimmer of hope and a sense of solidarity.

As Olivia navigated the challenges of treatment and recovery, she found solace in the stories of fellow survivors and members of the breast cancer community. Their shared experiences and collective resilience served as a beacon of hope, illuminating the path forward with strength and determination.

"I am continually inspired by the incredible strength and resilience of the breast cancer community," Olivia shared in a heartfelt message of gratitude. "Your stories of courage and perseverance have lifted me up on the darkest of days, reminding me that I am never alone in this fight."

Indeed, the breast cancer community is a testament to the power of resilience and solidarity in the face of adversity. From support groups to online forums, survivors and their loved ones come together to share their stories, offer words of encouragement, and uplift one another in times of need.

"To my fellow warriors, I want you to know that you are not alone," Olivia's message continued. "Together, we are stronger than cancer. Let us stand shoulder to shoulder, united in our fight, and never lose sight of the hope that lies within each and every one of us."

In the midst of darkness, there is always light. In the depths of despair, there is always hope. As Olivia Munn's journey through breast cancer has taught us, the power of love, support, and resilience knows no bounds. With each heartfelt message of hope and gratitude, we are reminded of the strength that resides within us all, guiding us through the darkest of times and illuminating the path forward with unwavering courage and grace.

Conclusion: A Call to Action

In concluding our journey through the experiences of Olivia Munn and the broader landscape of breast cancer awareness and advocacy, it's essential to reiterate the critical messages and call upon readers to take action in the fight against breast cancer.

Early detection stands as the cornerstone of effective breast cancer management. Olivia Munn's story underscores the importance of routine screenings and proactive healthcare. As she exemplified, a simple mammogram can be the catalyst for early intervention, potentially saving lives and offering more treatment options. Therefore, I implore each reader to prioritize their health by scheduling regular screenings and consultations with healthcare providers. By staying vigilant and proactive, we can detect breast cancer in its early stages when treatment outcomes are often more favorable.

Equally crucial is the support network surrounding individuals affected by breast cancer. Whether it's offering a listening ear, providing practical assistance, or participating in advocacy efforts, support from friends, family, and the community can make a profound difference in the journey toward healing and resilience. Let us commit to being compassionate allies to those navigating the challenges of breast cancer, offering unwavering support and understanding throughout their journey.

Furthermore, I urge readers to become active participants in raising awareness about breast cancer and supporting research and advocacy initiatives. By sharing personal stories, we not only break down stigmas and misconceptions but also foster a sense of solidarity within the breast cancer community. Every narrative shared adds to the collective voice advocating for improved healthcare access, better treatment options, and ultimately, a cure for breast cancer. Together, we can amplify awareness, dispel myths, and empower individuals to take charge of their breast health.

Moreover, supporting breast cancer research and advocacy efforts is paramount in driving progress toward better prevention, detection, and treatment methods. Whether through donations, volunteer work, or participation in fundraising events, each contribution plays a vital role in advancing scientific understanding and improving outcomes for those affected by breast cancer. Let us unite in our commitment to supporting organizations dedicated to breast cancer research, patient support, and advocacy, ensuring that no one faces this disease alone.

Finally, it's essential to express profound gratitude to Olivia Munn for her courage, transparency, and advocacy in sharing her breast cancer journey with the world. By bravely opening up about her experiences, she has not only inspired countless individuals but also catalyzed important conversations surrounding breast health, early detection, and resilience in the face of adversity. Olivia's unwavering strength and determination serve as a beacon of hope for those navigating similar challenges, reminding us all of the power of resilience and the importance of community support.

In closing, let us heed the call to action embedded within Olivia Munn's story and the broader discourse on breast cancer awareness and advocacy. Together, through early detection, proactive healthcare, support networks, advocacy efforts, and gratitude for those who lead by example, we can work towards a future where breast cancer is no longer a threat to the lives and well-being of individuals and their loved ones.

Made in United States
Orlando, FL
03 October 2024